The Easy Acid Reflux Diet Cookbook

Delicious Recipes for Taming Your Tummy and Savoring Life

EMMANUEL AKINNODI

TABLE OF CONTENTS

17. Grilled Shrimp Skewers

18. Sesame Ginger Broccoli

19. Baked Sweet Potato Fries

20. Tofu and Veggie Stir-Fry

21. Peach and Basil Salad

22. Stuffed Bell Peppers

23. Cucumber and Mint Infused Water

24. Baked Apples with Cinnamon

25. Chocolate Chia Pudding

14-DAY MEAL PLAN

CONCLUSION

INTRODUCTION

Step into the world of "The Easy Acid Reflux Diet Cookbook: Delicious Recipes for Taming Your Tummy and Savoring Life," where you'll find the ultimate culinary guide for alleviating acid reflux while indulging in mouthwatering meals.

Living with acid reflux can be tough, affecting not only our diets but also our enjoyment of food. But fret not! This thoughtfully curated collection of delectable recipes is here to make your journey to better digestive health a delightful experience.

Each recipe is gentle on your stomach yet bursting with flavors that will leave you craving for more. Say goodbye to bland dishes, as we prove that an acid reflux-friendly diet can still be delicious. Whether you're a seasoned cook or a kitchen novice, our easy-to-follow recipes empower you to take charge of your diet and well-being.

Within the book, you'll find a wide variety of dishes, from comforting breakfasts to satisfying lunches, mouthwatering dinners, and indulgent desserts. Within the book, you'll find not only a wide variety of delicious recipes but also a crafted out meal plan. This comprehensive meal plan is designed to be gentle on your stomach and cater to your specific dietary needs, ensuring you can make informed choices about your meals without the hassle of calculating nutritional information for each recipe. With this meal plan at your disposal, you'll be empowered to savor every bite while taking care of your tummy and enjoying the journey to better digestive health.

This cookbook isn't just about quick fixes; it's a lifestyle guide for individuals seeking a holistic approach to managing acid reflux. As you embark on this transformative journey, you'll discover the profound connection between food, mind, and body. By nurturing your well-being through wholesome and flavorful meals, you'll find yourself savoring not only the cuisine but also the moments that life has to offer.

So, let's embark on this flavorful journey together. Experience the joys of eating without the fear of discomfort, and let "The Easy Acid Reflux Diet Cookbook" be your trusted companion to a happier, healthier, and more flavorful life. Get ready to savor every delicious bite, one recipe at a time!

25 QUICK, EASY AND DELICIOUS ACID REFLUX RECIPES

1. Baked Almond-Crusted Chicken

Ingredients:

4 boneless, skinless chicken breasts

1 cup almond flour

1 teaspoon paprika

1 teaspoon garlic powder

Salt and pepper to taste

Preparation:

Preheat oven to 375°F (190°C).

Mix almond flour, paprika, garlic powder, salt, and pepper in a shallow bowl.

Coat chicken breasts in the almond flour mixture and place on a baking sheet.

Bake for 20-25 minutes until chicken is cooked through and golden brown.

2. *Quinoa and Roasted Vegetable Salad*

Ingredients:

1 cup cooked quinoa

1 cup of mixed roasted veggies, including cherry tomatoes, bell peppers, and zucchini

2 tablespoons extra virgin olive oil

1 tablespoon balsamic vinegar

Salt and pepper to taste

Preparation:

Toss cooked quinoa and roasted vegetables together in a bowl.

Drizzle with olive oil and balsamic vinegar, season with salt and pepper.

Mix well and serve.

3. Ginger and Turmeric Smoothie

Ingredients:

1 cup almond milk

1 ripe banana

1-inch piece of fresh ginger, peeled

1 teaspoon ground turmeric

1 tablespoon honey

Preparation:

Effortlessly merge all the ingredients into a harmonious blend, culminating in a lusciously smooth and creamy texture that will tantalize your taste buds.

Customize the sweetness to your liking by incorporating the delightful essence of honey, should your palate yearn for an extra touch of nectarous perfection.

Stir in the soy sauce and cook for another minute.

4. Salmon with Lemon-Dill Sauce

Ingredients:

4 salmon fillets

1/4 cup plain yogurt

1 tablespoon fresh dill, chopped

1 teaspoon lemon zest

Salt and pepper to taste

Preparation:

Season salmon with salt and pepper and grill or bake until cooked through.

Mix yogurt, dill, and lemon zest to make the sauce.

Serve salmon with the lemon-dill sauce on top.

5. Cauliflower Rice Stir-Fry

Ingredients:

1 head of grated cauliflower, prepared like rice

1 cup mixed veggies, including corn, peas, and carrots

2 tablespoons low-sodium soy sauce

1 tablespoon sesame oil

Preparation:

In a large skillet, sauté the grated cauliflower and mixed vegetables in sesame oil until tender.

Infuse the dish with the umami goodness of soy sauce, gently stirring it in, and allowing it to simmer and meld its flavors for just one more minute, bringing out a delightful depth to your culinary creation.

6. Baked Turkey Meatballs

Ingredients:

1 pound ground turkey

1/4 cup breadcrumbs (gluten-free, if preferred)

1 egg

1 teaspoon dried oregano

1 teaspoon garlic powder

Salt and pepper to taste

Preparation:

Preheat oven to 375°F (190°C).

Thoroughly blend the ingredients in a mixing bowl until they come together harmoniously.

Form the mixture into meatballs and arrange them neatly on a baking sheet.

Allow the meatballs to bake in the oven for 15-20 minutes until they are fully cooked.

7. Greek Yogurt Parfait

Ingredients:

1 cup plain Greek yogurt

1/2 cup mixed berries (blueberries, strawberries)

2 tablespoons honey

2 tablespoons chopped walnuts

Preparation:

In a glass, layer Greek yogurt, mixed berries, honey, and chopped walnuts.

Replicate the layers of the dish and serve it delightfully chilled.

8. Spinach and Feta Stuffed Chicken

Ingredients:

4 boneless, skinless chicken breasts

1 cup fresh spinach, chopped

1/2 cup crumbled feta cheese

1 tablespoon olive oil

Salt and pepper to taste

Preparation:

Preheat oven to 375°F (190°C).

Cut a pocket into each chicken breast.

Stuff with chopped spinach and feta cheese.

Season with salt and pepper.

In a skillet, heat up some olive oil over medium-high heat.

Carefully brown both sides of the chicken by searing it to perfection.

Transfer to the oven and bake for 15-20 minutes until chicken is cooked through.

9. Roasted Asparagus with Lemon

Ingredients:

1 bunch asparagus, trimmed

2 tablespoons olive oil

1 teaspoon lemon zest

Salt and pepper to taste

Preparation:

Preheat oven to 400°F (200°C).

Give the asparagus a lovely coating of olive oil, lemon zest, salt, and pepper.

Roast in the oven for 10-12 minutes until tender-crisp.

10. Mango and Avocado Salsa

Ingredients:

1 ripe mango, diced

1 avocado, diced

1/4 cup red onion, finely chopped

1 tablespoon fresh cilantro, chopped

1 tablespoon lime juice

Salt and pepper to taste

Preparation:

Gather all the components in a bowl to create a scrumptious combination.
 Season with salt and pepper.

Serve as a refreshing topping for grilled chicken or fish.

11. Brown Rice and Black Bean Burrito Bowl

Ingredients:

1 cup cooked brown rice

1 can of washed and drained black beans

1/2 cup diced tomatoes

1/4 cup chopped green onions

1/4 cup chopped cilantro

1 tablespoon lime juice

1/2 avocado, sliced

Preparation:

Mix brown rice, black beans, diced tomatoes, green onions, cilantro, and lime juice in a bowl.

Top with sliced avocado.

12. Baked Cod with Herbs

Ingredients:

4 cod fillets

1 tablespoon olive oil

1 teaspoon dried thyme

1 teaspoon dried rosemary

1 teaspoon dried parsley

Salt and pepper to taste

Preparation:

Preheat oven to 400°F (200°C).

Rub cod fillets with olive oil and sprinkle with dried herbs, salt, and pepper.

Bake for 12-15 minutes until fish flakes easily with a fork.

13. Zucchini Noodles with Pesto

Ingredients:

2 medium zucchinis, spiralized into noodles

1/4 cup fresh basil leaves

1/4 cup pine nuts

1/4 cup grated Parmesan cheese

1 clove garlic

1/4 cup olive oil

Salt and pepper to taste

Preparation:

In a food processor, blend basil, pine nuts, Parmesan cheese, garlic, olive oil, salt, and pepper until smooth.

Toss zucchini noodles with the pesto sauce.

14. Tuna and White Bean Salad

Ingredients:

1 can tuna, drained

1 can of washed and drained white beans

1/4 cup diced red onion

2 tablespoons chopped parsley

2 tablespoons lemon juice

2 tablespoons olive oil

Salt and pepper to taste

Preparation:

Mix tuna, white beans, red onion, parsley, lemon juice, olive oil, salt, and pepper in a bowl.

Serve as a refreshing salad on a bed of mixed greens or as a filling for a whole-grain wrap.

15. Eggplant and Tomato Stacks

Ingredients:

1 large eggplant, sliced into rounds

2 large tomatoes, sliced

1/4 cup fresh mozzarella, sliced

2 tablespoons balsamic glaze

Fresh basil leaves for garnish

Preparation:

Preheat oven to 375°F (190°C).

Place eggplant rounds on a baking sheet and bake for 10 minutes until softened.

Layer each eggplant round with a slice of tomato and mozzarella.

Drizzle with balsamic glaze and return to the oven for another 5 minutes until cheese is melted.

Just before serving, adorn the muffins with delightful fresh basil leaves for an extra touch of flavor and appeal.

16. Blueberry Oat Muffins

Ingredients:

1 cup rolled oats

1 cup almond milk

1 ripe banana, mashed

1/4 cup honey

1 teaspoon vanilla extract

1 cup blueberries

Preparation:

Preheat oven to 375°F (190°C).

In a bowl, mix rolled oats and almond milk.

Add mashed banana, honey, and vanilla extract, stirring until combined.
Gently fold in blueberries.

Portion the mixture evenly into a muffin tin that has been prepared with muffin cups.

Allow the bake to continue for 20-25 minutes, or until a lovely golden brown hue is achieved and the muffins are fully cooked.

17. Grilled Shrimp Skewers

Ingredients:

1 pound of peeled and deveined big shrimp

2 tablespoons olive oil

1 tablespoon lemon juice

1 teaspoon paprika

1 teaspoon garlic powder

Salt and pepper to taste

Preparation:

In a bowl, mix shrimp with olive oil, lemon juice, paprika, garlic powder, salt, and pepper.

Thread shrimp onto skewers.

Grill for 2-3 minutes on each side until shrimp are opaque and cooked through.

18. Sesame Ginger Broccoli

Ingredients:

2 cups broccoli florets

1 tablespoon sesame oil

1 tablespoon soy sauce

1 teaspoon fresh ginger, grated

1 teaspoon sesame seeds

Preparation:

In a skillet, sauté broccoli in sesame oil until tender-crisp.

Stir in soy sauce, grated ginger, and sesame seeds.

Cook for another minute before serving.

19. Baked Sweet Potato Fries

Ingredients:

2 big sweet potatoes, thinly sliced

2 tablespoons olive oil

1 teaspoon paprika

1/2 teaspoon garlic powder

Salt and pepper to taste

Preparation:

Preheat oven to 425°F (220°C).

Toss sweet potato strips with olive oil, paprika, garlic powder, salt, and pepper.

Spread them in a single layer on a baking sheet.

Let them bake until they turn crispy and beautifully golden, usually around 20-25 minutes.

20. Tofu and Veggie Stir-Fry

Ingredients:

1 block firm tofu, cubed

2 cups mixed vegetables (broccoli, bell peppers, snow peas)

2 tablespoons low-sodium soy sauce

1 tablespoon hoisin sauce

1 tablespoon vegetable oil

Preparation:

In a large skillet, sauté tofu cubes in vegetable oil until golden brown.

Take your favorite assortment of mixed vegetables and stir-fry them until they reach a tender, delightful state.

Then, blend in a perfect combination of soy sauce and hoisin sauce for an explosion of flavors.

Enjoy the savory goodness of the stir-fry by serving it over wholesome brown rice or quinoa, creating a wholesome and satisfying meal.

21. Peach and Basil Salad

Ingredients:

2 ripe peaches, sliced

1 cup fresh mozzarella balls

1/4 cup fresh basil leaves

2 tablespoons balsamic glaze

Preparation:

Arrange peach slices, mozzarella balls, and basil leaves on a plate.

Enhance the dish's appeal with a final touch – drizzle some luscious balsamic glaze over it before serving, adding a touch of tangy sweetness to every bite.

22. Stuffed Bell Peppers

Ingredients:

4 bell peppers, halved and seeded

1 cup cooked quinoa

1 can of washed and drained black beans

1 cup diced tomatoes

1/2 cup chopped red onion

1 teaspoon chili powder

1 teaspoon cumin

Salt and pepper to taste

Preparation:

Preheat oven to 375°F (190°C).

In a bowl, mix cooked quinoa, black beans, diced tomatoes, red onion, chili powder, cumin, salt, and pepper.

For a more filling option, fill bell pepper halves with the delectable quinoa mixture, turning them into flavorful and colorful stuffed peppers.

Roast the bell peppers in the oven for 20-25 minutes until they become tender.

23. Cucumber and Mint Infused Water

Ingredients:

1 cucumber, thinly sliced

10-12 fresh mint leaves

1 liter water

Preparation:

In a pitcher, add cucumber slices and mint leaves.

Fill the pitcher with water.

Allow the dish to chill in the refrigerator for a few hours prior to serving.

24. Baked Apples with Cinnamon

Ingredients:

4 apples, cored and halved

2 tablespoons honey

1 teaspoon ground cinnamon

Preparation:

Preheat oven to 375°F (190°C).

Place apple halves on a baking sheet.

Enhance the flavors by drizzling honey and sprinkling ground cinnamon over the prepared dish.

Bake for 15-20 minutes until apples are soft and caramelized.

25. Chocolate Chia Pudding

Ingredients:

1/4 cup chia seeds

1 cup almond milk

2 tablespoons cocoa powder

1 tablespoon honey

Preparation:

Create a chia seed-infused almond milk mixture by combining them in a jar.

Stir in cocoa powder and honey.

Refrigerate overnight or for at least 4 hours until the mixture thickens and forms a pudding-like consistency.

Indulge in a delightful selection of quick, simple, and mouthwatering recipes from the Acid Reflux Diet Cookbook. These dishes not only bring you nourishment and joy but also help in managing acid reflux effectively.

14-DAY MEAL PLAN

Day 1:

Breakfast: Ginger and Turmeric Smoothie
Lunch: Quinoa and Roasted Vegetable Salad
Dinner: Baked Almond-Crusted Chicken with Steamed Asparagus

Day 2:

Breakfast: Blueberry Oat Muffins with Sliced Peaches
Lunch: Tuna and White Bean Salad
Dinner: Eggplant and Tomato Stacks with Brown Rice

Day 3:

Breakfast: Chia Pudding with Sliced Banana and Walnuts
Lunch: Spinach and Feta Stuffed Chicken with Steamed Broccoli
Dinner: Baked Cod with Herbs and Quinoa Pilaf

Day 4:

Breakfast: Peach and Basil Salad with a dollop of Greek Yogurt
Lunch: Zucchini Noodles with Pesto and Cherry Tomatoes

Dinner: Baked Sweet Potato Fries with Grilled Shrimp Skewers

Day 5:

Breakfast: Mango and Avocado Salsa with Rice Cakes
Lunch: Stuffed Bell Peppers with a side of Mixed Greens
Dinner: Sesame Ginger Broccoli with Tofu and Veggie Stir-Fry

Day 6:

Breakfast: Baked Apples with Cinnamon and a drizzle of Honey
Lunch: Mediterranean Chickpea Salad
Dinner: Salmon with Lemon-Dill Sauce and Roasted Asparagus

Day 7:

Breakfast: Banana Almond Smoothie
Lunch: Greek Salad with Lemon-Dill Grilled Salmon
Dinner: Cauliflower Rice Stir-Fry with Baked Turkey Meatballs

Day 8:

Breakfast: Ginger and Turmeric Smoothie
Lunch: Quinoa and Roasted Vegetable Salad
Dinner: Eggplant and Tomato Stacks with Brown Rice

Day 9:

Breakfast: Blueberry Oat Muffins with Sliced Peaches
Lunch: Tuna and White Bean Salad
Dinner: Baked Cod with Herbs and Quinoa Pilaf

Day 10:

Breakfast: Chia Pudding with Sliced Banana and Walnuts
Lunch: Spinach and Feta Stuffed Chicken with Steamed Broccoli
Dinner: Baked Sweet Potato Fries with Grilled Shrimp Skewers

Day 11:

Breakfast: Peach and Basil Salad with a dollop of Greek Yogurt
Lunch: Zucchini Noodles with Pesto and Cherry Tomatoes
Dinner: Sesame Ginger Broccoli with Tofu and Veggie Stir-Fry

Day 12:

Breakfast: Mango and Avocado Salsa with Rice Cakes
Lunch: Stuffed Bell Peppers with a side of Mixed Greens
Dinner: Salmon with Lemon-Dill Sauce and Roasted Asparagus

Day 13:

Breakfast: Baked Apples with Cinnamon and a drizzle of Honey

Lunch: Mediterranean Chickpea Salad

Dinner: Cauliflower Rice Stir-Fry with Baked Turkey Meatballs

Day 14:

Breakfast: Banana Almond Smoothie

Lunch: Greek Salad with Lemon-Dill Grilled Salmon

Dinner: Quinoa and Roasted Vegetable Salad

You have the flexibility to either follow the meal plan provided or mix and match the recipes according to your personal preference. Enjoy your delightful gastronomic adventure with these acid reflux-friendly dishes!

CONCLUSION

In the captivating pages of the Acid Reflux Diet Cookbook, we embark on a transformative journey—one that extends beyond culinary delights. Throughout these recipes, we've uncovered the art of balancing a specialized diet practically and emotionally, finding relief and comfort in each carefully crafted combination of flavors.

Beyond a mere cookbook, this collection is a testament to the human spirit's strength and resilience in overcoming challenges. It pays tribute to those who have faced acid reflux, seeking solace in cooking and sharing meals with loved ones.

As we conclude this enchanting journey, let us remember that true healing lies not just in recipes but within ourselves. Armed with knowledge and compassion, we have the power to forge a path to a life free from acid reflux's burden.

May the knowledge gleaned here be a beacon of hope for all struggling with this condition, empowering us to savor every bite with gratitude. Amidst the challenges, we find light in the joy of creating nourishing meals.

As we bid farewell to this cookbook, may its impact resonate in our hearts, inspiring us to embrace our vulnerabilities and discover strength through healing.

May this mark the beginning of a new chapter—a chapter of resilience, wellness, and a profound connection to the essence of life. Each meal we share becomes an expression of love and self-care, transforming not just our bodies, but our souls.

With the wisdom from these pages, let us forge a path of wellness and healing, celebrating the triumph of the human spirit and the ability to rewrite our stories.

And so, with a heart full of gratitude and a spirit ignited with hope, let us set forth, not only to overcome the challenges of acid reflux but to savor every aspect of life's vibrant tapestry. May this be a journey of resilience, restoration, and renewal, where the transformative power of food and emotion intertwines to create a life that is truly worth savoring.